CBD-Rich Hemp Oil

Cannabis Medicine is Back

Dear Dick,

To your health!

Tina Rappaport

Steven Leonard Johnson

Authors

Tina Rappaport, BFA

Steven Leonard-Johnson, RN, PhD

Dedication

American Cannabis Nurses Association

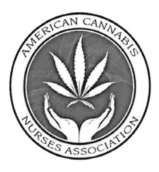

The medical world is changing and it is changing very quickly. Medical professionals can be hard pressed at times to keep pace. There are decisions to be made where to put one's time and energy while knowing what's important to investigate, research and study.

It is counterintuitive to put one's time and energy towards learning about certain plants, even though medicinal, if the plants are deemed illegal. MARIJUANA falls into this category. My nursing education did not include the medicinal benefits of MARIJUANA, with the exception of a medication named Marinol, a synthetic THC pharmaceutical, primarily used to treat the nausea and vomiting side effects of chemotherapy.

The American Cannabis Nurses Association was conceived by Ed Glick in 2006. By the year 2010, a colleague of his, Mary Lynn Mathre, MSN, RN joined forces with him and together they co-founded the American Cannabis Nurses Association (ACNA). The ACNA was formed to bring nurses together, to share, integrate and one day certify nurses in the science of endocannabinoid therapeutics nursing.[1]

Medical MARIJUANA has been prescribed to an estimated two and a half million people in 19 U.S. states as of 2012. Medical MARIJUANA is here, and it is here to stay. There is no going back. For this reason, it is important for all of the components of the cannabis plant to be considered, understood and studied. Although prescription cannabis is what most people have heard about, there is also a therapeutic component of the cannabis plant called cannabidiol (CBD), that can be purchased over the counter without a prescription. This needs to be included in our cannabis education. This book is to that aim. Although CBD is not psychoactive like THC and does not need a prescription to purchase the way medical cannabis does, it is still a component of the cannabis plant and used therapeutically. It is important for nurses to know and understand about all of the remedies a person takes, whether it is prescriptive or over the counter.

10 percent of the proceeds of this book

will be donated to the

American Cannabis Nurses Association

to help further their cause.

Dedication Reference:

[1] American Cannabis Nurses Association website: http://americancannabisnursesassociation.org

Table of Contents

FORWARD

Dr. Steven Leonard-Johnson, RN, PhD

The health benefits of cannabidiol (CBD) from the HEMP FAMILY of plants is this book's primary focus. To a lesser degree, the similarities and differences between HEMP and cannabis will also be explored. There is often much confusion between the two. A comprehensive understanding of both as they pertain to health and the unique medicinal value they each provide is presented.

Cannabis as medicine is not a new concept. Prior to prohibition, major pharmaceutical companies produced a wide variety of cannabis-based medicines and 1840 to 1937 were considered the "golden age" for cannabis medicine. In addition, cannabis has been used as a medicine for thousands of years dating back 1000 years BC in India and 5000 years BC in China, at least.

Although cannabis has a long history, what is new is the recent discovery (1992) of the body's endocannabinoid system (ECS). Also discovered was that the cannabis plant is loaded with phytocannabinoids (plant cannabinoids) that can stimulate the ECS receptor sites of this system. It is this combined discovery that is leading cannabis, in all forms, back into the limelight again as a viable medicine.

The facts speak for themselves, as many people are voting cannabis back into their lives. With the rapid changes sweeping the country pertaining to medical MARIJUANA legalization, it is incumbent for health care providers to learn about cannabis therapeutics and keep pace with the number of medical MARIJUANA prescriptions written and CBD over-the-counter use. Indeed, as with any other medication, health care providers must be educated about cannabis, as well as the anatomy and physiology of the endocannabinoid system.

With the relatively recent discovery of the endocannabinoid system, there has been a lag in the health care education system integrating ECS science into the curriculum. This book is presented as an initial study into this new science for both the professional and non-healthcare professional.

This book's goal is to bring the neophyte in cannabis therapeutics up to speed and provide a working knowledge in the area of cannabis therapeutics, which includes CBD.

We would also like to acknowledge and thank Dr.

Allen Frankel, MD of the Greenbridge Medical Services in Santa Monica, California. He has been a specialist in cannabis medicine for nearly a decade and generously shares his knowledge on his internet site and by issuing his educational seminars on YouTube. His website and YouTube sites are listed in the References.

DISCLAIMER

Please note that the information in this book is for educational purposes only and is not meant as an alternative to medical diagnosis or treatment. The authors make no representations or warranties in relation to the health information in this book. If you think you may be suffering from any medical condition, you should seek medical attention. You should never delay seeking medical advice, disregard medical advice, or discontinue medical treatment because of information in this book. If you are considering making any changes to your lifestyle, diet or nutrition, you should consult with your doctor.

These statements have not been evaluated by the Food and Drug Administration (FDA).

This information is not intended to diagnose, treat, cure or prevent any disease.

CHAPTER 1

Clearing the Confusion
Between Industrial Hemp and Marijuana

There can be much confusion around the classification of HEMP and cannabis. Below is an attempt to clarify their similarities and differences. The chart below will help explain their biological classifications.

Biological Classifications of Marijuana		
Category	Latin Name	Common Name
Kingdom	Plantae	Plants
Subkingdom	Tracheobionta	Vascular plants
Superdivision	Spermatophyta	Seed plants
Division	Magnoliophyta	Flowering plants
Class	Magnoliopsida	Dicotyledons
Subclass	Hamamelididae	None
Order	Urticales	None
Family	Cannabaceae	Hemp family
Genus	Cannabis L.	hemp
Species	Cannabis sativa L.	marijuana
Subspecies	Cannabis sativa L. ssp. Sativa	marijuana/sativa
Subspecies	Cannabis sativa L. ssp.indica	marijuana/indica
Subspecies	Cannabis sativa L. ssp. Ruderalis	marijuana/ruderalis

MARIJUANA and HEMP (also known as Industrial Hemp) both belong to the same plant family known as **HEMP FAMILY**, or *Cannabaceae* in Latin.

Under the **HEMP FAMILY**, they are both in the Genus **HEMP**, or *Cannabis L* in Latin.[1] Therefore, technically, "**cannabis**" refers to what is known as all types of MARIJUANA and HEMP.

This HEMP Genus of flowering plants includes a single Species commonly called **MARIJUANA** or *Cannabis sativa L* in Latin.

This Species of MARIJUANA has three further subspecies: MARIJUANA SATIVA (*Cannabis sativa L ssp. sativa*), MARIJUANA INDICA (*Cannabis sativa L ssp. indica*) and MARIJUANA RUDERALIS (*Cannabis sativa L ssp. ruderalis*).

For the purposes of this book, the following terms are used for clarification:

> **Cannabis**: to mean the entire HEMP FAMILY of plants.
>
> **MARIJUANA:** to mean the psychoactive varieties containing over 0.3% THC.
>
> **HEMP:** to mean the non-psychoactive CBD-rich plants containing below 0.3% THC.

HEMP

Scientifically, HEMP is the common name for plants of the entire Genus. *Cannabis L* is the Latin name as seen on the chart above. In non-scientific terms, HEMP is commonly used to refer only to the Cannabis strains traditionally cultivated for industrial use and not medicinal use. HEMP, or Industrial Hemp, is an extremely versatile plant used in manufacturing thousands of commercial products and more recently is being cultivated for its high CBD medicinal properties.[2]

HEMP, (*Cannabis L*) known as common HEMP is the variety grown for industrial use in Europe, Canada, and elsewhere. *Cannabis sativa L subsp. ruderalis*, usually has very low amounts of THC often less than 1% and is generally not used for medicinal and recreational purposes, however it may be a good source for CBD extract.

As of this writing, HEMP that is allowed to be grown legally in the United States falls under the Schedule 1 drug policy and enforcement of the U.S. because it contains some amounts of THC. If CBD oil was extracted from U.S. HEMP, it would not be allowed to be sold in the U.S. Any CBD oil that is sold in the U.S. must be imported from other countries.

MARIJUANA (the "pot" subspecies of *sativa* and *indica*) generally has poor fiber quality, but high THC content, and is primarily used for recreational and medicinal drugs. The major difference between HEMP and these MARIJUANA subspecies is the plant appearance and the amount of THC secreted in a resinous mixture by epidermal hairs called glandular trichomes. Strains of HEMP approved for Industrial Hemp produce only trace amounts of the psychoactive drug THC. Typically, HEMP contains below 0.3% THC, while MARIJUANA typically contains anywhere from 6 - 20% or more of THC.

It is important to understand that the HEMP FAMILY of plants has approximately 500 compounds, consisting of about 100 phytocannabinoids (THC and CBD are two), 120 terpenoids and many flavonoids to name the more prominent compounds in the cannabis plants.

HEMP Derived Cannabidiol (CBD)

The non-psychoactive cannabinoid called cannabidiol (CBD) has direct influence on bodily functions. This aspect will be addressed in subsequent chapters. CBD can be extracted from the Industrial Hemp plant. There is a growing movement in America and around the world that promotes the use of the CBD phytocannabinoid for health benefits. CBD is sold commercially and it is a very safe substance.

Commercial CBD products have a THC content below 0.3%, not enough of a concentration to produce a high. Cannabis plants (all species in the HEMP FAMILY) have varying ratios of THC to CBD and these are the most important ratios when prescribing medical MARIJUANA for a known condition. Certain ratios work better with a specific illness and are prescribed accordingly. High CBD with below 0.3% THC preparations can conveniently be purchased without a doctor's prescription and they are legal in every state.

These CBD-rich products range from liquid HEMP oil, HEMP oil as a thick paste, oil in capsules, sublingual tincture drops or sprays, salves for topical use, edibles as in candy or gum and CBD vapor from vaporizers similar to e-cigarettes. The list of CBD-rich products will surely expand over time.

Chapter 1 References:

[1] Wikipedia:
http://en.wikipedia.org/wiki/Cannabaceae

[2] HEMPATHETICS: What is Industrial Hemp?
http://hempethics.weebly.com/what-is-industrial-hemp.html

CHAPTER 2

Understanding the Importance
of the Endocannabinoid System

The first cannabinoid was discovered in 1964 by Dr. Raphael Mechoulam, PhD. Dr Mechoulam was a professor of medicinal chemistry and natural products at Hebrew University in Jerusalem, Israel. He was the first to synthesize the cannabinoid Tetrahydrocannabinol (THC).

Three decades later, in 1992, Dr. Mechoulam made another important discovery. Dr. Mechoulam and his team identified anandamide, a naturally occurring human neurotransmitter. Anandamide was named after the Sanskrit word ananda, which means "bliss" or "delight". Anandamide, also known as N-arachidonoylethanolamine or AEA, is an endogenous cannabinoid neurotransmitter (the word endogenous means it is produced within the body). The discovery of the neurotransmitter anandamide led to the subsequent discovery of the endocannabinoid system.

Hence, in 1992, the newly discovered endocannabinoid system was named for the cannabis plant from which Dr. Mechoulam synthesized the first THC back in 1964.

The endocannabinoid system is composed of receptor sites and endogenous endocannabinoids throughout the body. This widespread system is found in the brain, organs, glands, connective tissue and immune cells and it has regulatory roles in many physiological processes including appetite, pain-sensation, mood and memory. The primary purpose of this system revolves around maintaining balance in the body; this is known as homeostasis.

What is a Cannabinoid?

There are three general types of cannabinoids. The first type is the one produced in our own body known as "endogenous cannibinoids". The second type is produced by plants and is called "phytocannabinoids". The third type is synthetically engineered in a lab and is known as "synthetic cannabinoids".

Regardless of type, cannabinoids act as

neuromodulators and help regulate every physiological system such as our nervous system, digestive system, reproductive system, immune system, endocrine system, and muscular system. Cannabinoids are an essential component involved in keeping the body systems balanced and stable, maintaining what's known as homeostatic balance.[1]

Our focus will be the plant derived cannabinoid, or phytocannabinoid, called CBD (cannabidiol). CBD is extracted from the HEMP plant, is becoming hugely popular in the marketplace, and, it deserves a closer look.

Receptor Sites
of the Endocannabinoid System (ECS)

Cannabinoid receptor sites are found throughout the entire body, embedded in the membrane of the cell. They act as lock-and-key-like chemical receptors. The cannabinoids have signals to which the receptors respond. The receptors receive the cannabinoids. This system is estimated to be over 600 million years old and is found in all vertebrate species. We are just finding out about it now and just beginning to understand how widespread and important it is to our functioning.

There are two primary receptor sites of mention when working with phytocannabinoids. The two types are cannabinoid receptors CB1 and CB2. These two receptor sites have been identified and are found in the nervous system as well as the peripheral tissues and organs. These were discovered in 2003.

There are additional receptor sites throughout the human body that respond to plant compounds. The cannabis family of plants are not the only plants that have compounds that can bond to human receptor sites. Let's mention several other instances where plant substances other than phytocannabinoids find a place to bind in the human body.

One well-known plant substance that binds to a human receptor site is opium. This substance is found in the poppy plant. Another example of a human receptor site bonding with a plant substance is tobacco. Nicotinic receptors in the brain that normally bind with acetylcholine will bind with nicotine instead. Whereas nicotine and opium can be highly addictive, there is much less of a potential of addiction and severe withdrawal with MARIJUANA. It is theorized that acute withdrawal from THC is mitigated by the fact that

THC is stored in the fat cells of the body and has a time release factor, slowly releasing THC into the system for longer periods, thereby lessening withdrawal effects.

In the past ten years, the endocannabinoid system has been shown to be involved in a growing number of physiological functions in both the organs and in the central and peripheral nervous systems. Researchers are finding out that by modulating the endocannabinoid system a number of diseases and pathological conditions may be alleviated. Conditions such as multiple sclerosis, cancer, stroke, obesity/metabolic syndrome, anxiety disorders, neuropathic pain, Huntington's disease, myocardial infarction, movement disorders, hypertension, glaucoma, seizure disorders, Parkinson's and osteoporosis are a sampling of the diseases helped and there are many more.

Human breast milk and the cannabis plants have something in common - some of the same cannabinoids. Breast milk is abundant in cannabinoids. These similar cannabinoids protect the infant against disease, stimulate the suckling response and help to regulate the appetite. Cannabinoid levels in the body are nutrition dependent, whereas the levels drop with poor nutrition, i.e. lack of Omega-3 oils.

The **cannabinoid receptor type 1**, often abbreviated as **CB$_1$**, is a G protein-coupled cannabinoid receptor located primarily in the central and peripheral nervous system. It is activated by the endocannabinoid neurotransmitters anandamide and 2-arachidonoyl glyceride (2-AG); by plant cannabinoids, such as the compound THC, an active ingredient of the psychoactive drug cannabis; and by synthetic analogues of binol.[2]

The **cannabinoid receptor type 2**, abbreviated as **CB$_2$**, a G protein-coupled receptor from the cannabinoid receptor family that in humans is encoded by the *CNR2* gene. It is closely related to the cannabinoid receptor type 1, which is largely responsible for the efficacy of endocannabinoid-mediated presynaptic-inhibition, the psychoactive properties of tetrahydrocannabinol (THC), the active agent in MARIJUANA, and other phytocannabinoids (natural cannabinoids). The principal endogenous ligand for the CB$_2$ receptor is 2-arachidonoylglycerol (2-AG).[3]

The above explanation of CB1 and CB2 receptors may seem a bit complex. There is a very deep rabbit hole of intricate biochemical processes involved with the CB receptors. This book will not address that overwhelming complexity - it will be kept simple.

To simplify this for a basic understanding, let's break it down. The CB1 and CB2 receptors have the job of helping to regulate hormone and neuro-hormone activity. The fundamental function of the CB1 and CB2 receptors is either to "excite" or to "inhibit". This excite or inhibit process will determine how other hormones and body systems are regulated in the body.

The endocannabinoid system is fundamentally a hormone regulation system throughout the body and it helps to keep the body in balance. Consequently, it is easy to see how the minutiae of so many physiological systems may rely on the ECS. There is much yet to be learned about this system. The role of receptor stimulation of the major phytocannabinoids CBD, THC and CBN is addressed in Chapter 3.

Nutrition and Endocannabinoid Production in the Body

We would be remiss if this important nutritional fact was omitted. Omega-3 fatty acids are the precursor for the body to produce its own endocannabinoids. Let's not lose sight of the fact that the body has been making its own endocannabinoids for hundreds of millions of years and it does so with fatty acids. Some of the literature is now suggesting that a diet deficient in Omega-3 fatty acids can destabilize behavior and a diet deficient in Omega-3 fatty acids can deform or break our CB1 receptors on brain cells. Hence, our nutrition, once again, is of prime importance.

It is prudent to try the least invasive, safest therapies first and work up the ladder. It makes sense that the cannabinoids produced in our own bodies are enough and are the best available.

If our body systems were optimally functioning, including the endocannabinoid system, then a diet rich in Omega-3 fatty acids would serve us well, as these fatty acids are the nutritional precursor the body uses to make its own endocannabinoids. We were designed to make our own, but endocannabinoid production is nutrition dependent. Good diet, exercise and staying well hydrated are also very important components to health that must be considered. The body wasn't designed to need an external source of cannabinoids if it was producing enough of its own. However, our 21st century diets are often less than optimal.

Omega-3 fatty acids help repair and grow CB1 receptors and the CB1 receptors cannot work properly if starved of Omega-3s. It would be very helpful for anyone using a cannabis preparation (or not) to incorporate Omega-3 fatty acids into the diet, priming the CB1 receptors to be at their best for endocannabinoids or phytocannabinoids. Regular inclusion of foods high in omega-3 fatty acids is a good overall strategy.

Omega-3 fatty acids are needed to help keep our brain cells healthy in general. Omega-3 fatty acids are the brain-boosting, cholesterol-clearing good fats. They are good for your joints, skin, vision, brain, heart, cholesterol levels and even boosts fertility. Omega 3's are anti-aging and an anti-inflammatory. Consider some of the benefits of Omega-3 fatty acids that dovetail with the ECS:

Omega-3 fatty acids:

- Lubricate joints to avoid wear and tear, hence less pain and less inflammation

- Fights wrinkles by making our skin's third layer thicker and smoother.

- Protects vision, as our eyes' health is dependent on the liver (who knew?). The liver helps metabolize fat-soluble vitamins that feed and maintain the eye's membranes.

- Maintains a healthy heart since Omega 3s reduce triglycerides, stabilize your heartbeat, make platelets "less sticky" and can even lower blood pressure.

- Attacks acne - an inadequate intake of omega-3 fatty acids contributes to breakout-prone skin.

- Clears cholesterol while boosting levels of HDL (the good cholesterol) and helps clear your arteries.

- Boosts the brain by altering your neurotransmitters to help reduce depression.

- Improves fertility rates in both males and females by improving sperm's swimming ability and the environment for implantation in women.

- Pregnancy prerequisite, Omega-3 fatty acids directly affect brain development, making it crucial for expectant mothers. When the mother doesn't have enough of these essential fatty acids, the baby borrows from her.

Omega-3s are found naturally in a variety of delicious foods including walnuts, flaxseeds, chia seeds, sardines, salmon, tuna, fresh basil, spinach, beans, Brussels sprouts, cauliflower, broccoli and avocados to get you started.

It seems that it would be far better, to be at the maximum natural production of cannabinoids and be able to internally make enough supply to meet our demands than to be dependent on an external supply.

However, there are many reasons why the body may not meet its endocannabinoid demands. Experiencing an acute or chronic stressor or multiple stressors, systemic compromise such as genetic or digestive issues, the demands and alterations of emotional and physical trauma, pollution and buildup of internal toxins are situations that could change the supply and demand needs for endocannabinoids.

Many well-known conditions can develop in the body that might require supplementation. For instance, the hormonal system may not function properly, as in people with diabetes, and a person may require insulin; the nervous system may be firing excessively causing acute or chronic pain necessitating a pain medication; perhaps the gastrointestinal system has the inability to metabolize Vitamin B12 necessitating B12 injections. Likewise, it stands to reason that people suffering from a cannabinoid deficiency also be given what they need to relieve their suffering and the chance to function in a healthy way.

The cannabis family of plants is our only option for a natural, organic phytocannabinoid medicinal.

Chapter 2 References:

[1] CannabinoidSociety.com:
http://cannabinoidsociety.com/about/what-is-cbd/

[2] Wikipedia: Cannabinoid receptor type 1
http://en.wikipedia.org/wiki/Cannabinoid_receptor_1

[3] Wikipedia Cannabinoid receptor type 2
http://en.wikipedia.org/wiki/Cannabinoid_receptor_type_2

CHAPTER 3

Distinction Between Medical Marijuana and the Single Phyto-Cannabinoid CBD

Tetrahydrocannabinol (THC)　　　Cannabidiol (CBD)

Cannabis

As one can see in the diagram above, THC and CBD have the same molecular formula, but are a bit different structurally. CBD is basically a structural isomer of THC. It is this slight difference in structure between the two that enables THC to produce a "high" in the user, and CBD to not.

Both CBD and THC are found in HEMP and MARIJUANA in differing ratios. THC and other identified cannabinoids CBD, CBN, CBG, CBC and dozens more, are phytocannabinoids produced through photosynthesis in hair-like trichomes on the surface of the cannabis plant during the flowering phase.[1]

The different Species of cannabis plants have a wide variety of ratios of THC to CBD. For instance, *Cannabis sativa L ssp. sativa* can have a THC:CBD ratio 4-5 times that of *Cannabis sativa L ssp. indica*, meaning sativa strains have high levels of THC and comparatively low levels of CBD. It is now common to grow the strains that best suit one's needs. For example, one commercial strain of medicinal cannabis can have a 41:1 ratio of THC:CBD and another commercial cannabis medicinal may have a 0.42:1 THC:CBD ratio. *Cannabis sativa L ssp. ruderalis* is generally low in THC and is typically not used for medicinal preparations. This information is important to note, as all medications can produce unwanted side effects and cannabis is no different, due to THC.

There are 120 or so aromatic terpenoids in cannabis plants that give cannabis its distinctive scent when burned. Many researchers are of the opinion that these terpenoids have a direct and synergistic therapeutic effect with the cannabinoids and other compounds of the plant. A whole plant compound will be treated more as a food by the body than will a synthetic compound and will metabolize differently as well.

Therefore, there is a general consensus of many prescribers and users that believe the synthetic forms of the cannabinoid molecule will not be as effective as direct extracts from the cannabis plant itself.

Although THC is often prescribed to mitigate the side effects of other treatments, such as the nausea and vomiting caused by chemotherapy, THC in and of itself can cause some unwanted side effects (anxiety, schizophrenia, etc.). CBD has been shown to reduce the intense "high" side effect of THC, as well as the THC side effects of altered consciousness, confusion and anxiety.[1]

For the people needing the therapeutic benefits of THC, but not being able to handle the unwanted side effects of it, strains of cannabis with a higher CBD to THC ratio are indicated.

There are many challenges ahead for cannabis therapeutics. A Schedule 1 classification like the one listed below makes it very difficult to conduct research on the same scale as a non-scheduled substance. The laws are stringent in that cannabis has a Schedule 1 drug classification, as follows:

Schedule 1 Drug Classification:

Schedule 1 drugs, substances, or chemicals are defined

as drugs with no current accepted medical use and a high potential for abuse. Schedule 1 drugs are the most dangerous drugs of all the drug schedules with potentially severe psychological or physical dependence. Some examples of substances listed in Schedule 1 are: heroin, lysergic acid diethylamide (LSD), marijuana (cannabis), peyote, methaqualone and 3,4-methylenedioxymethamphetamine ("Ecstasy").[2]

With the onset of some states legalizing medical MARIJUANA and the plethora of reports that it helps so many people with a wide range of conditions, the above drug classification may one day, hopefully in the near future, be recognized as having medicinal value.

Cannabis as a Pharmaceutical

Another challenge for the cannabis plant, beside its classification, is that the plants grow as they will, without any kind of perfect or exact, repeatable combination or ratio of their components. One of the reasons cannabis was dropped from the U.S. Pharmacopeia back in the early 1940's was in part because of its uniformity problems, as every batch would be slightly or more than slightly different. Prescribing a medicine is difficult when the property of the medicine changes from bottle to bottle and batch to batch.

As cannabis slowly gains acceptance city by city and state by state across America, which is definitely happening, it remains to be seen how it will unfold, as American medicine is firmly grounded in the precision synthetic pharmaceutical model. Precision medications offer a sense of safety to both the person administering and the person receiving.

However, it is the other 483 compounds in cannabis, the ones that many practitioners feel are synergistically important such as the cannabinoids, terpenes and flavonoids to name a few, where exact measurements in the finished product become a challenge. If it were only the THC and CBD molecules, as in a synthetic, it would be a simple matter to analyze and consistently reproduce.

On the other hand, humans have been using cannabis preparations successfully for thousands of years, in spite of it not being an exact science. Many practitioners are more than willing to work with the variable organic compounds in cannabis, as they are not always uniform.

Nonetheless, cannabis physicians and nurses, pioneers really, seem to be learning as they go given the variable cannabis extracts. These doctors seem quite knowledgeable about the components of the cannabis extracts they are working with and have turned it into an art form when prescribing with them. It remains to be seen how cannabis preparations, both with the THC and/or CBD, will fit in to the pharmaceutical model.

Then again, maybe it remains to be seen how the pharmaceutical model will fit into the cannabis plant model. American physicians are used to highly accurate medicines and the cannabis plant extracts coming to market may defy this model.

The Legal Phytocannabinoid Cannabidiol (CBD)

CBD, from HEMP, can be purchased in the United States simply by ordering it online, legally. After importation, the CBD rich oil is analyzed for purity and processed further before it is sold as a dietary supplement. CBD is not psychoactive and is considered safe for over the counter type use for a wide range of conditions. CBD products may contain trace amounts of THC, below 0.3%, but this amount is not enough to be psychoactive, or get one high. Although HEMP is not grown in the U.S., except under certain conditions, it is legal to import HEMP-based products into the U.S. and CBD rich oil is one of the products allowed.

Government studies have proven CBD to be a very safe product. In the wording of a patent held by The U.S. Department of Human Services, US Patent #66,30,507, it states the following:

"No signs of toxicity or serious side effects have been observed following chronic administration of cannabidiol to healthy volunteers (Cunha et al., Pharmacology 21:175-185, 1980), even in large acute doses of 700 mg/day (Consroe et al., Pharmacol. Biochem. Behav. 40:701-708, 1991)"

The patent also states the following:

US Government Patent #6,630,507:
"Cannabinoids as Antioxidants & Neuroprotectants"

Key points in the government patent on CBD:

1. This patent recognizes CBD's ability as an anti-epileptic, which means its anti-seizure.

2. CBD has powerful antioxidant activity that can be used in the prophylaxis and treatment of oxidative associated diseases. Some of the conditions generally thought to be correlated with oxidative stress are Alzheimer's disease, Parkinson's disease, cancer and autism.

3. CBD has ability to lower intraocular pressure in the treatment of glaucoma.

4. CBD is protective to the brain from ischemic damage (helping blood and oxygen flow).

5. CBD is a naturally occurring constituent, hence cannabinoid of the HEMP plant and according to US government patent #6,630,507 it supports the nutritional health of aging bodies.

6. CBD has an anxiolytic effect, which means anti-anxiety.

7. CBD has neuro-protective properties, which means it protects the cells of the nervous system, the brain and nerves in the body.

8. CBD has the ability to protect against cellular damage.

9. CBD does not have toxicity issues or serious side effects in large acute doses.

In Summary

Cannabis therapeutics is an emerging health science. Obviously, in the past, there was little, if any, education around the cannabis plant both in nursing and medical schools. Now, however, there is a growing need for more nurses and healthcare providers to step up to the plate and help educate one another about this emerging science. There are now Continuing Education Credit courses for doctors and nurses, and one can only hope that cannabis therapeutic education will be included in formal healthcare curriculum going forward.

The road ahead may be a little rocky because of the controversy surrounding use of medicinal cannabis, but even some major pharmaceutical companies have recently filed patents for their synthetic cannabinoids and claim a host of diseases their synthetic cannabinoids will help. Synthetic cannabinoids may lack the full array of compounds found in the cannabis plant, but synthetic cannabinoids will be far easier to maintain quality control and they can be patented, which is appealing to these companies.

One must wonder, however, if there was profit to be made from whole plant compounds in terms of patents, such as with Sativex, would big Pharma have more interest in developing whole plant medicinals? The rocky road lies ahead in that MARIJUANA is still a scheduled drug, it is a plant that cannot be patented and its compounds are complex to replicate in a laboratory.

As the endocannabinoid system is a major regulatory system in the body, it makes sense, and is most humane, to develop and provide medications that work with this system in an effort to relieve suffering caused by a malfunctioning or deficiency. It is important to note that although we are proponents of the whole plant medicine, when dealing with extremely ill patients with delicate systems, psychiatrically or physically, medicinal accuracy counts more than ever. Therefore, nothing is off the table here. There is a place for whole plant synergy and there is a place for precise pharmaceutical accuracy in dosing with the extremely ill patient.

How many natural options are there really?

The only plants known to contain cannabinoids enough to treat the endocannabinoid system are found in the HEMP FAMILY plants.

Chapter 3 References:

[1] The Human Solution:
http://the-human-solution.org/education-resources/education/cannabis/the-endocannabinoid-system/

[2]) US Drug Enforcement Agency website:
http://www.justice.gov/dea/druginfo/ds.shtml

CHAPTER 4

Your Endocannabinoid System
May Be Deficient

Most of us believe eating well, drinking good water, getting adequate exercise, taking vitamins and managing stress are good ideas for being healthy. We might even throw in additional supplements, like resveratrol, extra B vitamins, fish oils or even curcumin. We make the leap of faith that these things will protect our health.

If you're reading this book, there's a strong likelihood that your good habits have not been enough and maybe your health has turned out to be less than optimal. Perhaps it's diabetes, cancer, arthritis, fibromyalgia, heart disease, psoriasis, obesity, osteoporosis, IBS, depression, anxiety, insomnia or an arm's-length list of other ailments that's got you down.

You're searching for answers and you're not alone.

With the relatively recent discovery of your body's Endocannabinoid System (ECS) approximately 20 years ago, cannabinoids and their related compounds from cannabis plants are showing widespread benefits throughout your body.

Cannabidiol is "a cannabinoid devoid of psychoactive effect,"[1] and may have broad clinical potential for an astonishing spectrum of ailments. CBD has been shown, in clinical settings, to help relieve convulsions, inflammation, anxiety, nausea, and other health concerns; in fact, hundreds of peer-reviewed studies indicate that CBD possesses almost unbelievable clinical potential. A literature review from 2009 recapped CBD's documented capabilities as an anxiolytic (anti-anxiety), antipsychotic, antiepileptic, neuroprotectant, vasorelaxant (lower blood pressure), antispasmodic, anti-ischemic, anti-cancer agent, antiemetic, antibacterial agent, anti-diabetic, anti-inflammatory, and even as a means to stimulate bone growth.[2] CBD has also been shown to strengthen and improve the efficiency of mitochondria, the "powerhouses" of your cells that are responsible for ensuring that your cells work the way they should.[3]

Medical MARIJUANA and CBD (cannabidiol) research is currently accelerating and there are indications that your system, your endocannabinoid system (ECS), may very well be deficient. Some researchers have hypothesized that your ECS may function better with supplementation and the benefits may be profound and widespread. It appears your ECS has the enormous job of regulating a myriad of metabolic processes from cell death (as in cancer) to bone growth (as in osteoporosis), from anxiety to autoimmune disorders, from pain to pregnancy.

There are several VERY BASIC "cannabis" type strains to consider with differing THC to CBD ratios – remember that they are all members of the "HEMP FAMILY" and different species are now being bred for varying ratios. Each species has its own palette of terpenes, other co-factors and are suitable for alleviating different conditions.

1. **High THC to low CBD ratio** - Common "MARIJUANA" (pot) generally used recreationally and medicinally.

2. **Closer to 1:1 THC to CBD ratio** – MARIJUANA used medicinally and for patients who are too reactive to high THC strains.

3. **Low THC to High CBD ratio** – Not as common, this MARIJUANA is used therapeutically. This is the "Charlotte's Web" type of MARIJUANA (1:24 THC to CBD ratio), preferred for seizure disorders and is subject to states' MARIJUANA laws.

4. **High CBD to below 0.3% THC ratio** – Known as "Industrial Hemp", the oil is extracted for therapeutic benefits. This will not get you high. This is where our focus will be, as it is readily available, legal in all 50 states and no prescription is necessary.

When you poke around on the internet, you find many sites saying

CBD is :   Anti-cancer

Anti-bacterial

Anti-inflammatory

Anti-anxiety

Anti-oxidant

And CBD: Regulates blood sugar

Promotes bone growth

Suppresses muscle spasm

Reduces seizures

Relieves pain

Reduces autoimmune response

And more. If research proves this true, and there's plenty of indications it is, CBD could be the ultimate over-the-counter nutritional supplement. CBD-rich HEMP oil, the essential oil of the HEMP plant, has over 480 natural compounds including 100 or so cannabinoids (CBD and THC are two) and over 120 terpenes (limonene like in lemons is one) along with amino acids, proteins, enzymes, ketones, fatty acids, steroids, flavonoids, vitamins and more. The term "CBD" has come to mean this whole plant extract high in Cannabidiol (CBD) with much smaller amounts of the other compounds.

Although there are synthetic cannabinoid substances produced by pharmaceutical companies, it is believed that the naturally occurring plant substances (**phyto-**cannabinoids) act synergistically, known as the "Entourage Effect", for optimal benefits.

Clinical
Endocannabinoid Deficiency Syndrome
(CEDC)

You may be surprised to know that mother's milk provides endocannabinoids, and we go on to produce our own, throughout our lifetime. If we are not producing them adequately, our Endocannabinoid System (ECS) cannot function properly, resulting in Endocannabinoid Deficiency Syndrome as first suggested by Dr. Ethan Russo in 2004. Dr. Russo concludes, "migraine, fibromyalgia, IBS and related conditions display common clinical, biochemical and pathophysiological patterns that suggest an underlying clinical **endocannabinoid deficiency** that may be suitably treated with cannabinoid medicines."[4]

"In the past decade, the endocannabinoid system has been implicated in a growing number of physiological functions, both in the central and peripheral nervous systems and in peripheral organs... modulating the activity of the endocannabinoid system turned out to hold therapeutic promise in a wide range of disparate diseases and pathological conditions, ranging from mood and anxiety disorders, movement disorders such as Parkinson's and Huntington's disease, neuropathic pain, multiple sclerosis and spinal cord injury, to cancer, atherosclerosis, myocardial infarction, stroke, hypertension, glaucoma, obesity/metabolic syndrome, and osteoporosis, to name just a few…"[5]

Since the endocannabinoid system (ECS) regulates numerous physiological functions, **CEDC** may be the underlying cause for the myriad of conditions CBD seems to help. Phytocannabinoids bind to the ECS in the same way as our own "endo"cannabinoids, making for excellent supplementation. Phytocannabinoid (CBD) supplementation may be both a powerful disease preventative and a homeostasis restorative.

Dr. Robert Melamede has a Ph.D. in Molecular Biology and Biochemistry from the City University of New York and is retired as Chairman of the Biology Department at University of Colorado in Colorado Springs where he continues to teach and research cannabinoids, cancer, and DNA repair. Dr. Melamede speculates that a healthy endocannabinoid system will minimize age-related illnesses:

> "People are generally aware that Omega-3's are good for you and they inhibit various cardio vascular problems. What most people are not aware of is that they

participate directly in the endocannabinoid system, in that they make a variety of our endocannabinoids, and they are part of the bigger picture of lipid metabolism of which the endocannabinoid system is kind of a central focal point. So there are numerous benefits from these essential fatty acids that we can help modulate, we can change our biochemistry, by our nutritional intake... So that for many, many, many people with a whole huge spectrum of illnesses, ranging from cardio vascular disease, skeletal disease like osteoporosis, cognitive dysfunction from neurological deterioration associated with aging, and literally all the auto-immune diseases, and many cancers, they all have free radicals as part of their ideology. And cannabinoids, be they the ones we make or the ones we take in, benefit those."[6]

We've all heard of free radicals as "the bad guys" responsible for aging and age-related illnesses and how anti-oxidants "scavenge" up the free radicals. Free radical creation is promoted by inflammation. CBD is known to inhibit inflammation so, in turn, CBD, with its anti-oxidant properties, may also have an inhibiting factor on free radicals, hence age-related diseases. These are exciting times, indeed.

Just consider these research studies:

- Researchers at the University of Milan in Naples, Italy reported in the *Journal of Pharmacology and Experimental Therapeutics* that non-psychoactive compounds in marijuana inhibited the growth of glioma cells in a dose-dependent manner, and selectively targeted and killed malignant cells through apoptosis (normal cell death). "**Non-psychoactive CBD (cannabidiol) produces a significant anti-tumor activity both in *vitro* and *in vivo*,** thus suggesting a possible application of CBD as an antineoplastic (tumor inhibiting) agent."[7]

- The first experiment documenting cannabinoid anti-tumor effects took place in 1974 at the Medical College of Virginia at the behest of the U.S. government. The results of that study, reported in an August 18, 1974 *Washington Post* newspaper feature, showed that marijuana "**slowed the growth of lung cancers, breast cancers and a virus-induced leukemia** in laboratory mice and prolonged their lives by as much as 36%."[8]

- Cannabis has been found to be effective in relieving the pain of rheumatoid arthritis.[9]

- Cannabidiol (CBD) arrested the onset of autoimmune diabetes in NOD (non-obese diabetes-prone) mice in a 2007 study.[10]

- In 2006, researchers at Hadassah University Hospital in Jerusalem[11] reported that injections of 5 mg per day of CBD (10-20 injections) significantly reduced the prevalence of diabetes in mice from an incidence of 86% in non-treated controls to an incidence of only 30%.

- And, from the National Cancer Institute's website[12], they summarize that preclinical studies of cannabinoids have investigated the following activities[13]:

Antitumor Activity

- Studies in mice and rats have shown that cannabinoids may inhibit tumor growth by causing cell death, blocking cell growth, and blocking the development of blood vessels needed by tumors to grow. Laboratory and animal studies have shown that cannabinoids may be able to kill cancer cells while protecting normal cells.

- A study in mice showed that cannabinoids may protect against inflammation of the colon and may have potential in reducing the risk of colon cancer, and possibly in its treatment.

- A laboratory study of delta-9-THC in hepatocellular carcinoma (liver cancer) cells showed that it damaged or killed the cancer cells. The same study of delta-9-THC in mouse models of liver cancer showed that it had antitumor effects. Delta-9-THC has been shown to cause these effects by acting on molecules that may also be found in non-small cell lung cancer cells and breast cancer cells.

- A laboratory study of cannabidiol in estrogen receptor positive and estrogen receptor negative breast cancer cells showed that it caused cancer cell death while having little effect on normal breast cells.

- A laboratory study of cannabidiol in human glioma cells showed that when given along with chemotherapy, cannabidiol might make chemotherapy more effective and increase cancer cell death without harming normal cells.

Stimulating Appetite

- Many animal studies have shown that delta-9THC and other cannabinoids stimulate appetite and can increase food intake.

Pain Relief

- Cannabinoid receptors (molecules that bind cannabinoids) have been studied in the brain, spinal cord, and nerve endings throughout the body to understand their roles in pain relief.

- Cannabinoids have been studied for anti-inflammatory effects that may play a role in pain relief.

More CBD Facts You Should Know

An interesting fact observed with CBD is that as time goes on, you need a lesser dose to achieve the same effects due to cannabinoids, like CBD (and THC), being fat-soluble compounds. Your body stores cannabinoids in fat, and gradually releases them so their effects are prolonged. This is why many cannabis users can fail (THC) drug tests days or weeks after ingesting or inhaling cannabis.

In an article published in The British Journal of Pharmacology by Dr. Ethan Russo (July 12, 2011), "Taming THC: Potential Cannabis Synergy and Phytocannabinoid-Terpenoid Entourage Effects", Russo discusses many, many potential uses for cannabinoid therapy including anti-inflammatory, analgesic, anti-cancer, antibiotic, antifungal, anti-nausea, anti-MRSA, anti-anxiety, memory protection and reduction of stroke risk.[14]

A-Pinene is just one of the many terpenes found in cannabis and is widely found in nature, particularly in conifer trees and the herb rosemary, and has an insect-repellant role. In humans it is anti-inflammatory and a bronchodilator and has been effective against MRSA. These terpenes, part of a plant's essential oils, contribute to a plant's scent, flavor and color and may have some therapeutic effects simply by aroma. Limonene is another well-known terpene and it is found in the yellow skin of lemons. Limonene is known to have anti-bacterial, anti-depressant and anti-carcinogenic properties.

All of the compounds found in the various Hemp Family of plants – the cannabinoids, the terpenes, the fatty acids, the enzymes, etc. – they all act together in a synergistic symphony (The Entourage Effect), each playing it's part to create the whole. This implies some beneficial functions may be lost if only one substance from the whole plant is teased out.

Research Documenting CBD Benefits

It has been reported that cannabinoids are promising medicines to slow down disease progression in neurodegenerative disorders including Parkinson's, Alzheimer's and Huntington's.

Evidence suggests that cannabis shows benefit for the prevention and treatment of Alzheimer's disease and an Australian research team, led by Dr. Tim Karl, suggests that CBD can help reverse some of the cognitive effects associated with Alzheimer's. After using Cannabidiol (CBD) on mice suffering from memory loss, the researchers found that the mice showed signs of regaining their cognitive abilities. The conclusion was that Cannabidiol could successfully treat neurodegenerative diseases like Alzheimer's, Parkinson's and Huntington's. Explaining his team's results to The Sydney Morning Herald, Dr. Karl had the following to say, "It basically brings the performance of the animals back to the level of healthy animals. You could say it cured them." Cannabidiol (CBD) helps in neurogenesis, which is the generation of new neurons in the hippocampus area of the brain – this is the part where memory is formed, organized, and stored. Neurons play a central role in the transmission of messages not only within the brain but also throughout the nervous system. [15] [16] [17]

You may be asking what other illnesses might researchers think CBD would be of benefit?

More to the point, might CBD help me?

Following is a small, partial list of studies (Kindle version is hyperlinked) to consider. You're encouraged to do further research, keeping the ratio of CBD to THC in mind, and paying attention to what compound the researchers attribute benefits. The list below is an attempt to include research focusing primarily on Cannabidiol (CBD), as it is readily available and legal in every state.

Acne:

ECS of the Skin and Cannabidiol as a Treatment for Acne.
www.ncbi.nlm.nih.gov/pubmed/19608284
www.beyondthc.com/wp-content/uploads/2013/08/CBD-for-Acne.pdf

Anxiety:

CBD significantly reduces anxiety and SAD (Social anxiety Disorder).
www.jop.sagepub.com/content/25/1/121.short
www.ncbi.nlm.nih.gov/pmc/articles/PMC3079847/

Arthritis - Osteoarthritis Pain:

Studies show the widespread endocannabinoid system likely plays a role in the regulation of pain, inflammation and joint function.
www.ncbi.nlm.nih.gov/pubmed/24494687

Arthritis - Rheumatoid Arthritis, Types 1 and 2 Diabetes, Atherosclerosis, Alzheimer Disease, Hypertension, the Metabolic Syndrome, Ischemia-reperfusion Injury, Depression, and Neuropathic Pain:

Cannabidiol's potential in targeting oxidative stress in various diseases.
www.ncbi.nlm.nih.gov/pubmed/21238581

Arthritis:

CBD offers protection of the joints against severe damage.

www.pnas.org/content/97/17/9561.full

Cancer:

In 2012, researchers at the California Pacific Medical Center in San Francisco found CBD could stop metastasis in breast, brain, prostate and other aggressive cancers.

www.online.wsj.com/article/PR-CO-20130528-906109.html

Cancer:

Cannabinoids - anti-tumor, programmed cell death, appetite stimulation and pain.

www.cancer.gov/cancertopics/pdq/cam/cannabis/healthprofessi onal/page4

Cancer – Prostate:

Cancer cells have more cannabinoid receptors sites than healthy cells.

www.jbc.org/content/281/51/39480.long

Colon:

Cannabinoid system is physiologically involved in the protection against excessive inflammation in the colon.

www.ncbi.nlm.nih.gov/pmc/articles/PMC385396

LDL Formation:

Cannabidiol is a potentially useful therapeutic agent for treatment of atherosclerosis.
www.ncbi.nlm.nih.gov/pubmed/21804214

MRSA & Antibacterial Action:

All five major cannabinoids show potent activity against MRSA.
www.ncbi.nlm.nih.gov/pubmed/18681481

Neurodegenerative Disorders (i.e., Alzheimer's, Parkinson's, Huntington's):

New clinical applications for Cannabidiol.
www.ncbi.nlm.nih.gov/pubmed/22625422

Niemann-Pick Disease:

Cannabidiol may relieve symptoms.
www.ncbi.nlm.nih.gov/pubmed/6732800

Obesity & Metabolic Syndrome:

Endocannabinoid-modulatory anti-obesity therapeutics may also help metabolic syndrome, diabetes type-2, atherothrombosis, inflammation, and immune disorders.
www.ncbi.nlm.nih.gov/pmc/articles/PMC3681125/

Osteoporosis:

British researchers show the endocannabinoid system plays an important role in regulation of bone mass

and CBD decreases bone resorption.
www.ncbi.nlm.nih.gov/pmc/articles/PMC3001217/
www.ncbi.nlm.nih.gov/pubmed/19070683

Pain:

Linking the Endocannabinoid System with modulation
of pain and inflammation.
www.ncbi.nlm.nih.gov/pmc/articles/PMC3820295/

Reproduction:

The Endocannabinoid System has a role in successful
fetus implantation and early pregnancy.
http://humupd.oxfordjournals.org/content/13/5/501.full.pdf

Schizophrenia:

Brazilian researchers conclude cannabinoids may be a
potential therapeutic strategy.
http://www.ncbi.nlm.nih.gov/pmc/articles/PMC3915876/

How do I take CBD and Where Can I Get it?

CBD-rich HEMP Oil comes in various concentrations
and forms: liquid HEMP oil, HEMP oil as a thick paste,
oil in capsules, sublingual tincture drops or sprays,
salves for topical use, edibles as in candy or gum and
CBD vapor from vaporizers similar to e-cigarettes. The
list of CBD-rich products will surely expand over time.

Products range in dose concentration, making it easy to choose a product that will provide maybe 1 mg of CBD, all the way up into hundreds of mgs. One such oil provides approximately 0.5 mgs per pump, while another provides three times that amount per pump. There are candies providing 5 mg each and capsules with 25 mgs.

Higher concentrated products include syringe dispensers for oil and paste. These concentrations range from about 15% to 25% CBD content, providing 150 - 250 mg per gram of oil. In the near future, some companies may come out with CBD with even higher concentrations.

These varying concentrations allow a person to start at a very low dosage, working up until the sought after effect is obtained. Keep in mind CBD can have a biphasic effect at higher doses. This means what is beneficial at a low dose, may have an undesirable effect at a high dose. More on this in the next chapter.

Personal preference and dosage desired will dictate which product you choose. The lowest amount comes in flavored oils, while the highest amount of CBD is available in a thick, resinous paste with a strong flavor that some find difficult. Of course this thick paste can be masked in things like applesauce or coconut oil and swallowed, but the most efficient way to ingest CBD oils is under the tongue (for 60-90 seconds) as much of the CBD is absorbed and then by-passes the digestive system.

As for how much CBD YOU should take? No suggestions for dosages will be made; however, reference to The Mayo Clinic's Marijuana Dosage Page [18] is included. Please note, however, that THC, CBD and pharmaceutical products are mentioned in this list.

As for where to get CBD-rich HEMP Oils? These products are sold on the internet and one must compare the CBD content in milligrams per serving to suit one's needs when choosing products for a particular condition. It is legal to ship and consume these products in all 50 states.

Readers of this book are eligible to receive a 10% discount on already discounted CBD product prices at www.URparamount.com – use coupon code "CBD10" at checkout.

Chapter 4 References:

[1] www.google.com/patents/US6630507

[2] www.ncbi.nlm.nih.gov/pubmed/19729208

[3]
www.rstb.royalsocietypublishing.org/content/367/1607/3326.
abstract?sid=20cf2c23-e4fd-49e3-9398-ec8be2e00226

[4] www.ncbi.nlm.nih.gov/pubmed/15159679

[5] www.ncbi.nlm.nih.gov/pmc/articles/PMC2241751/

[6]
www.archive.org/details/HolisticBiochemistryOfCannabinoi
ds-RobertMelamede

[7] Massi et al. 2004. Antitumor effects of cannabidiol, a non-
psychotropic cannabinoid, on human glioma cell lines.
Journal of Pharmacology and Experimental Therapeutics
Fast Forward 308: 838-845.

[8] www.alternet.org/drugreporter/20008

[9] www.medicalnewstoday.com/releases/33376.php

[10] www.ncbi.nlm.nih.gov/pmc/articles/PMC2270485

[11] Autoimmunity; 2006, Vol. 39, No. 2, Pages 143-151.

[12]
www.cancer.gov/cancertopics/pdq/cam/cannabis/patient/page2

[13]
www.cancer.gov/cancertopics/pdq/cam/cannabis/healthprof
essional/page4

[14] www.ncbi.nlm.nih.gov/pmc/articles/PMC3165946/

[15]
www.informahealthcare.com/doi/abs/10.1517/14728222.2012.
671812

[16]
www.link.springer.com/article/10.1007%2Fs00213-014-3478-5

[17]
www.journal.frontiersin.org/Journal/10.3389/fncel.2013.0001
8/full

[18]
www.mayoclinic.org/drugs-
supplements/marijuana/dosing/hrb-20059701

CHAPTER 5

The Wide Therapeutic Scope of CBD

The information set forth is informational only and is not meant to be prescriptive in any way. The following information is from studies and anecdotal reports of people who have tried CBD.

Many pharmaceutical companies have already produced a few synthetic cannabinoids and will no doubt produce many more, but many professionals remain of the opinion that whole plant extracts will always be superior for working in the body in a whole food, holistic, organic manner. It is this "Entourage Effect" that has so many doctors and health professionals convinced that whole plant extracts are more beneficial when taking supplemental cannabinoids

This being said, in the world of medicine where accuracy will always be appreciated, synthetics have some desirable advantages in production and predictability in dosing over plant extracts, but there may be a price to pay in forgoing the organic richness of the plant extract. The cannabis plant cannot be patented, obviously a drawback to the big pharmaceutical firms and without big Pharma's interest in the "whole plant" extract, funding for research is harder to come by, since the drug companies fund much of our medical research.

It takes an enormous amount of time, energy and money to get a drug approved for commercial use in the U.S., but the cannabis plant is here now and is already being used. After all, cannabis has already been perfected by mother nature. Since the cannabis plant may not fit into the pharmaceutical model like other drugs, there may be a grass roots movement outside of big Pharma. So far, this seems to be what is happening given the amount of YouTube video testimonies and popularization of CBD from celebrities like CNN's Dr. Gupta.

In any event, you have to hand it to the cannabis plant. It has survived the onslaught of some of the most severe propaganda and laws, but it still shines through all the controversy.

Biphasic Properties of CBD

The phytocannabinoid CBD has biphasic properties. An example of a biphasic effect can be illustrated with the substance alcohol that also has biphasic properties. Alcohol has a stimulating effect (happy, uninhibited, and carefree) when consuming up to a blood alcohol level of 0.05%. When drinking past 0.05%, alcohol will then have a depressant effect, not a stimulating one.

Drinking more does not make you "happier". This is known as biphasic, when a substance produces one type of effect at a lower dose level of consumption and a different type of effect at an increased level of consumption and these effects are dose dependent. Cannabinoid compounds have biphasic properties whereby small doses and high doses have opposite effects.

Cannabidiol and Drug Interactions

Cannabidiol is metabolized in the liver by a system known as the cytochrome P-450 enzyme system. This system is responsible for metabolizing up to 90% of drugs.

If the cytochrome P-450 enzyme system is functioning normally and predictably, a drug will have a predictable life span in the system. In other words, a drug that is known to stay active in the system for 12 hours will be active in the system for just that, 12 hours.

The problem comes when multiple drugs are taken. Some medications can slow down drug metabolism and other medications can speed it up. If one medication slows it down, the other medications may accumulate within the body to toxic levels.[1] On the other hand, if a medication speeds up drug metabolism, it may effectively create a shortage of the intended medication level.

Cannabidiol can slow down some types of drug metabolism within the P450 enzyme system.[2] Other issues that can cause a compromised P-450 enzyme system can be genetic, or issues of body toxicity from pesticides and such that can damage this liver enzyme system.

It is important to understand that cannabidiol levels in the system are affected by the health of the liver and by the effects that other drugs we may be taking have on the liver. There are saliva tests available that can measure the health of the P-450 enzyme system.

Doctors will test this system so they know how much of a medication dose to give someone. They can increase the dose with a faster metabolism and lower the dose for a slower metabolism. The alterations in liver enzyme metabolism due to medication influences may be minimal, or they could be significant, but still worth noting as these interactions need to be considered.

If you are taking medications, ask your doctor how the medications you are on affect the cytochrome P-450 enzyme system. If you want to look for yourself, there is an excellent online resource called the Davis's Drug Guide: The Cytochrome P450 System: What Is It and Why Should I Care? Here you will find a very comprehensive list of medications that affect the liver P-450 enzyme system.[3]

Suggested Dose of CBD

One of the best qualities of CBD is that it is a very safe product. People have taken upwards of 750 mgs of synthetic CBD at a time in government testing situations and have had no serious side effects. If you have never taken a product before, it is always a good idea to start with a small amount, because we can never know if an allergy, intolerance or side effect may appear. The chances of an adverse reaction to CBD at lower amounts is a very low probability.

Dr. Allan Frankel, MD, a cannabis specialist, states that he has started people with a suggested 1 or 2 mgs of CBD taken orally. He goes on to say that it will normally last for about 12 hours. So 1 to 2 mgs seems to be a low-end starting dose and may very well end up being the dose. Some other people experienced in CBD dosages suggest that 4 to 8 mgs a day is a suggested general amount taken by people with mild conditions.

It is also important to consider that cannabinoids are stored in fat cells. One may not need as much after taking them for a while, a few weeks perhaps. Our individual metabolisms and needs must also be considered, as no two people are exactly alike.

The general rule when using CBD is to go "low and slow", meaning start off at a very low dose and increase slowly, preferably under a doctor's order. Some manufacturers sell 25 mg capsules of CBD, suggesting this amount is what some people might use. Other considerations besides metabolism and sensitivity are a person's weight, as a person's weight is sometimes factored in with dosing formulas.

As with any medication, it is always best to do it under the care of your health care provider. When taking cannabinoids, certain clinical areas need special consideration. Schizophrenia, anxiety disorders and anyone with a psychological consideration, should especially consider that cannabinoids, even over the counter ones like CBD, are best taken under the supervision of a health professional. In addition, when taking a higher dose of CBD for issues such as neuropathic pain, it is advisable to consult with your health care provider.

Promising Cannabidiol Research

The CB1 receptors are prominent in the brain and the CB2 receptors are prominent in the peripheral nervous system and immune system.

CBD (cannabidiol) does not directly "fit into" (bind) to the CB1 or CB2 receptor sites, as does THC (tetrahydrocannabinol) and CBN (cannabinol). THC primarily stimulates the CB1 receptors and CBN primarily stimulates the CB2 receptors. As stated, CBD does not directly "fit into" (bind) to either receptor, but it does have a stimulatory effect on both the CB1 and CB2receptors.

CBD does bind to some other "G-protein-coupled" receptors however. For example, CBD binds directly to the TRPV-1 receptor. This receptor is known to mediate inflammation, pain perception and body temperature. There is ongoing research into the therapeutic effects of CBD on these and other conditions.

Some other ways CBD indirectly affects the endocannabinoid system are as follows:

1. CBD inhibits the breakdown of the body's own natural cannabinoid anandamide, by suppressing the enzyme fatty acid amide hydroxylase (FAAH), the enzyme that breaks down anandamide. This is significant because it helps to preserve the body's natural cannabinoid, anandamide, and keeps it from being destroyed. This results in greater activation of the CB1 receptor by the anandamide, which in turn enhances the body's innate protective responses of the endocannabinoid system.

2. Another action of CBD is that it stimulates the release of another endocannabinoid called 2-AG, and this release also stimulates the CB1 and CB2 receptors.

3. CBD powerfully opposes the action of THC at the CB1 receptor, thereby muting the psychoactive effects of THC. This is valuable in therapy when the side effects of THC need to be eliminated. Ratios of 1:1 THC:CBD, or less, can be implemented, with very good therapeutic success, greatly reducing the psychoactive properties of the THC.

There is a great deal of current research, much of it sponsored by the government, indicating that CBD directly activates serotonin receptors causing an anti-depressant effect.

Some of the most exciting CBD research is showing a potent anti-tumor effect. In a pre-clinical study at the California Pacific Medical Center in San Francisco conducted by Dr. Sean McAllister, reports indicate CBD down-regulates a gene called the ID-1, a gene implicated in several types of aggressive cancers. CBD turns off the over-expression of the ID-1 gene. Cancers with a high profile of the ID-1 gene are the only cancers ID-1 works with and this does not include all cancerous tumors, but it does include aggressive, metastatic cells. High levels of these metastatic cells have been found in cancers like leukemia, pancreatic, ovarian, lung, brain cancers and other types of cancers.[4]

CBD has a low-toxicity profile and has down-regulate ID-1 expression in aggressive human breast cancer cells. For cancers that are ID-1 driven, CBD holds a lot of promise in killing the cancer cells. CBD is able to inhibit ID-1 expression at the mRNA and protein level in a concentration-dependent fashion.[4]

A pharmaceutical cannabis medication called Sativex is now on the market and it is a whole plant extract having a 1:1 ratio of THC and CBD. It has been approved in over 20 countries for the treatment of neuropathic pain and is under phase III clinical trials in the United States. It's taken by spraying it under the tongue, and it is produced by GW Pharmaceuticals, a British company.

In one study published by the Journal of Neuroscience titled, *"Cannabidiol, a nonpsychotropic component of cannabis, inhibits cue-induced heroin-seeking and normalizes discrete mesolimbic neuronal disturbances"*, the study showed that CBD may actually help prevent heroin cravings and relapse, because it lowered stimulus cue-induced heroin seeking behavior.[5]

In another study in the Journal of Neuroscience,

"Addictive Behaviors" a team of researchers from the University College London did a double blind study showing that a group of smokers given CBD had a "significant reduction in the number of cigarettes smoked without increased craving". This could not be said of the non-CBD control group.[6]

The following conditions on this comprehensive list either are in preclinical trials or have been reported by people that CBD had helped them with their afflictions:

Acne
ADD/ADHD
Addiction
AIDS
ALS (Lou Gehrig's Disease)
Alzheimer's
Anorexia
Antibiotic Resistance
Anxiety
Atherosclerosis
Arthritis
Asthma
Autism
Bipolar
Cancer
Colitis/Crohn's
Depression

Diabetes

Endocrine Disorders

Epilepsy/Seizure

Fibromyalgia

Glaucoma

Heart Disease

Huntington's

Inflammation

Irritable Bowel

Kidney Disease

Liver Disease

Metabolic Syndrome

Migraine

Mood Disorders

Motion Sickness

Multiple Sclerosis

Nausea

Neurodegeneration

Neuropathic Pain

Obesity

OCD

Osteoporosis

Parkinson's

Prion/Mad Cow Disease

PTSD

Rheumatism

Schizophrenia

Sickle Cell Anemia

Skin Conditions

Sleep Disorders
Spinal Cord Injury
Stress
Stroke/TBI

Chapter 5 References:

[1] www.en.wikipedia.org/wiki/Cytochrome_P450

[2] Potent inhibition of human cytochrome P450 3A isoforms by cannabidiol: role of phenolic hydroxyl groups in the resorcinol moiety. www.ncbi.nlm.nih.gov/pubmed/21356216

[3] Davis's Drug Guide: The Cytochrome P450 System: What Is It and Why Should I Care?
www.drugguide.com/ddo/ub/view/Davis-Drug-Guide/109519/all/The_Cytochrome_P450_System:_What_Is_I t_and_Why_Should_I_Care_

[4] Cannabidiol as a novel inhibitor of Id-1 gene expression in aggressive breast cancer cells.
www.ncbi.nlm.nih.gov/pubmed/18025276

[5] Cannabidiol, a nonpsychotropic component of cannabis, inhibits cue-induced heroin-seeking and normalizes discrete mesolimbic neuronal disturbances
www.ncbi.nlm.nih.gov/pmc/articles/PMC2829756/

[6] Cannabidiol reduces cigarette consumption in tobacco smokers: Preliminary findings.
www.cannabisclinicians.org/wp-content/uploads/2013/07/CBDcigarettes.pdf

CHAPTER 6

Addiction to Marijuana:
Let's Examine the Facts

Even though this book is primarily about CBD, I, Steve Leonard-Johnson, wanted to have my say about the need for medicinal MARIJUANA, voice my opinions and show my support for legalization.

As with many substances, plant based or not, legal or not, there can be the potential for addiction. Many pharmaceutical drugs being prescribed today can be highly addictive, whether they're synthetic or plant-based. I've worked in the field of addiction and recovery as a registered nurse and it was not uncommon for people to be in detox for an addiction to a benzodiazapine (anti-anxiety) medication or for a pain medication, no matter if the drug was legally prescribed or obtained on the street illegally.

Obviously, there is a risk/benefit associated with most medications. Even at the commercial level, it is well known that people can develop tolerances, addictions and/or withdrawal symptoms from accepted commodities such as the caffeine in coffee, the nicotine in cigarettes and from alcohol, yet these products are readily available. To some people food can be addictive. People can become addicted to many things that are readily available - it doesn't have to be an illicit drug or a pharmaceutical to have an addiction potential.

So can MARIJUANA be addictive? The truthful answer is yes, it can be addictive. I personally know people who are in recovery for MARIJUANA addiction. I've read estimates of around 11% (1 out of 9) of the people who use MARIJUANA will get addicted and the younger the individual the more detrimental it can be. The numbers vary depending on the source. There are also significant estimates of addiction to alcohol and cigarettes. As for CBD, it is non-toxic, legal, and non-addictive due to its below 0.3% THC content.

I have been working as an RN in the field of psychiatry and recovery for many years. Withdrawal from cannabis may not be as dramatic or life threatening as withdrawal from alcohol, but addiction to and withdrawal from cannabis is real and people definitely seek treatment. Many proponents of recreational MARIJUANA don't like to acknowledge cannabis addiction, because they think it will lessen the chance of getting MARIJUANA legalized. However, I feel a responsibility to mention my experience. It is a reality. So much so, the criteria of how addiction to cannabis is diagnosed is included below. This criteria is from the Diagnostic and Statistical Manual 5 (DSM 5) that psychiatrists use to make a psychiatric diagnosis.

The DSM-5 defines a substance use disorder as the presence of at least 2 of 11 criteria listed below in the rating scale, which are clustered in four groups.

> **Mild Addiction** - would be 2 to 3 symptoms from the indicators listed below.
>
> **Moderate Addiction** - would be 4 to 5 symptom from the indicators listed below
>
> **Severe Addiction** - would be 6 or more symptom from the indicators listed below.

A. *Impaired control*:

1. taking more or for longer than intended

2. unsuccessful efforts to stop or cut down use

3. spending a great deal of time obtaining, using, or recovering from use

4. craving for substance

B. *Social impairments:*

    5. failure to fulfill major obligations due to use

    6. continued use despite problems caused or exacerbated by use

    7. important activities given up or reduced because of substance use

C. *Risky use:*

    8. recurrent use in hazardous situations

    9. continued use despite physical or psychological problems that are caused or exacerbated by substance use

D. *Pharmacologic dependence:*

    10. tolerance to effects of the substance

    11. withdrawal symptoms when not using or using less[1]

Substance related disorders are classified into two groups: substance induced and substance use disorders. When cognitive, psychiatric, sleep or sexual dysfunction results from abusing a drug, it is known as Substance Induced Disorder. When someone continues to use a substance despite the continued problems it causes in their lives, it is known as Substance Use Disorder.

Many addictions can be the result of people medicating themselves, without seeking standard treatment for their issues. I've seen a great deal of people self medicate. Self-medicating is an attempt by an individual to use a substance in an effort to obtain relief from some form of discomfort. One can self-medicate with many things, coffee, cigarettes, alcohol, food, methamphetamine, heroin, and cannabis to name a few. For instance, someone might feel anxious, drink some alcohol and no longer feel anxious. When people self-medicate, often times they aren't even aware of it. Self-medicating, at best, if repeated often enough, may lead to an addiction, either psychological or physical.

Adverse side effects of MARIJUANA may include:

- Rapid beating of the heart
- Low blood pressure
- Muscle relaxation
- Bloodshot eyes
- Slowed digestion and movement of food by the stomach and intestines
- Dizziness
- Depression
- Hallucinations
- Paranoia [2]

Symptoms of withdrawal from MARIJUANA may include:

- Irritability
- Trouble sleeping
- Restlessness
- Hot flashes.
- Nausea and cramping (rarely occur)

These symptoms are mild compared to withdrawal from opiates and usually lessen after a few days.[2]

One of the problems with self-medicating is that people can get into a great deal of trouble. When people use street drugs and highly addictive drugs with no medicinal value (illegal drugs) to self-medicate, for example methamphetamine or heroin, they may feel good for a while, but they will inevitably end up with yet an additional problem of addiction on top of the problem they were trying to medicate. Self-medicating keeps people from getting the proper help they need for the original problem.

I can understand how someone would use MARIJUANA on their own to help themselves to self-medicate, given MARIJUANA's medicinal properties, however, it would still be self-medicating and one could still run the risk of the same problems self-medicating can create.

Certain addictions have an additional medical and/or life threatening concern. I.V. drug use is in this category. These last few years, it made quite an impression on me seeing how many young people are now addicted to heroin, meth and cocaine. I have had many conversations with these young patients and they all conveyed to me how easy it was to get hooked on hard drugs. We had one patient starting a meth habit at 12 years old and soon thereafter started to shoot meth I.V. by the time she was 14. The most disturbing part was that her friends didn't turn her on to meth. Her meth-addicted father was giving it to her.

This story is to drive home the point that MARIJUANA does not belong to the same category as highly addictive "scheduled drugs". Addictions to meth, heroin, cocaine, etc. are much more severe, destructive and difficult to undergo recovery.

I have seen many infectious diseases associated with I.V. drug use of meth and heroin, running the gamut of infected skin, abscesses at the needle site, hepatitis, HIV and other sexually transmitted diseases from various drug seeking activity. Other problems encountered with hard drug use were poor nutrition, assault and battery, criminality, serious legal issues, broken homes and homelessness to name some of the more prevalent issues associated with IV drug use.

The way the drug laws are currently, they are likely sending destructive messages to teenagers that the schedule 1 drug, MARIJUANA, is more addictive and dangerous than the Schedule 2 drugs of OxyContin or fentanyl.[3] The fact is however, that if they take too much of either fentanyl or OxyContin, it could be fatal via respiratory depression, closing down of the lungs. Respiratory depression cannot happen with cannabis.

Definition of Controlled Substance Schedules [3]

Drugs and other substances that are considered controlled substances under the Controlled Substances Act (CSA) are divided into five schedules. An updated and complete list of the schedules is published annually in Title 21 Code of Federal Regulations (C.F.R.) §§ 1308.11 through 1308.15[4]. Substances are placed in their respective schedules based on whether they have a currently accepted medical use in treatment in the United States, their relative abuse potential, and likelihood of causing dependence when abused. Some examples of the drugs in each schedule are listed below.

Schedule I Controlled Substances

Substances in this schedule have no currently accepted medical use in the United States, a lack of accepted safety for use under medical supervision and a high potential for abuse.

Some examples of substances listed in Schedule I are: heroin, lysergic acid diethylamide (LSD), Marijuana (cannabis), peyote, methaqualone and 3,4-methylenedioxymethamphetamine ("Ecstasy").

Schedule II/IIN Controlled Substances (2/2N)

Substances in this schedule have a high potential for abuse which may lead to severe psychological or physical dependence.

Examples of Schedule II narcotics include: hydromorphone (Dilaudid®), methadone (Dolophine®), meperidine (Demerol®), oxycodone (OxyContin®, Percocet®) and fentanyl (Sublimaze®, Duragesic®). Other Schedule II narcotics include: morphine, opium and codeine.

Examples of Schedule IIN stimulants include: amphetamine (Dexedrine®, Adderall®), methamphetamine (Desoxyn®) and methylphenidate (Ritalin®).

Other Schedule II substances include: amobarbital, glutethimide and pentobarbital.

Schedule III/IIIN Controlled Substances (3/3N)

Substances in this schedule have a potential for abuse less than substances in Schedules I or II and abuse may lead to moderate or low physical dependence or high psychological dependence.

Examples of Schedule III narcotics include: combination products containing less than 15 milligrams of hydrocodone per dosage unit (Vicodin®), products containing not more than 90 milligrams of codeine per dosage unit (Tylenol with Codeine®) and buprenorphine (Suboxone®).

Examples of Schedule IIIN non-narcotics include: benzphetamine (Didrex®), phendimetrazine, ketamine and anabolic steroids such as Depo®-Testosterone.

Schedule IV Controlled Substances

Substances in this schedule have a low potential for abuse relative to substances in Schedule III.

Examples of Schedule IV substances include: alprazolam (Xanax®), carisoprodol (Soma®), clonazepam (Klonopin®), clorazepate (Tranxene®), diazepam (Valium®), lorazepam (Ativan®), midazolam (Versed®), temazepam (Restoril®) and triazolam (Halcion®).

Schedule V Controlled Substances

Substances in this schedule have a low potential for abuse relative to substances listed in Schedule IV and consist primarily of preparations containing limited quantities of certain narcotics.

Examples of Schedule V substances include: cough preparations containing not more than 200 milligrams of codeine per 100 milliliters or per 100 grams (Robitussin AC®, Phenergan with Codeine®) and ezogabine.[3]

MARIJUANA may be abused more, but saying it is more addictive and dangerous than other scheduled drugs, is a premise that's hard to agree with. Perhaps a more accurate message about cannabis would be, yes, it can be addictive, so be responsible if you use it and don't abuse it, similar to the message for alcohol use. And, of course, MARIJUANA should be legalized for medicinal use, no question.

The strains of MARIJUANA out there today are many times more potent than what was smoked in the 1960s. Back then, the THC content, the psychoactive component of MARIJUANA, was around 1.5 to 3%. Now the potency of THC can range around 10% or higher, and there are strains available today approaching 27% and even higher. These higher THC strains are mostly responsible for much of the negative side effects that come from today's MARIJUANA.

The THC in MARIJUANA can cause some people to become extremely anxious and even have psychotic symptoms. CBD can help mitigate the THC effects, as it helps to neutralize the THC psychoactive component. Unfortunately, some strains of MARIJUANA have been bred to have a very high THC level and a very low CBD level for recreational purposes, and again, these are the strains that can cause the most negative side effects.

Legal MARIJUANA growers in Colorado, like the ones featured in Dr. Gupta's CNN special on medical MARIJUANA, are now cultivating MARIJUANA strains designed to yield very low THC levels and much higher than previous CBD levels. This ratio has been hugely successful in treating children with a severe seizure disorder called Dravet Syndrome, where a child may have 200+ seizures a week. After taking the CBD-rich MARIJUANA preparation, it is reported that seizures drastically reduced to perhaps one seizure a week – and this has been reported to help enough children that medical MARIJUANA access laws are changing fast. One MARIJUANA strain with low THC and high CBD has been labeled "Charlotte's Web", after the little girl, Charlotte, featured in Dr. Gupta's documentary, was helped tremendously by this special medical MARIJUANA plant.[5]

The goal of the Colorado MARIJUANA growers is to get the anti-seizure type MARIJUANA plants to an eventual 30:1 ratio of CBD to THC. It is the CBD that has the primary anti-seizure effects. The benefits of the rest of the plant components will still be in the medicine. It is important to point out that once a ratio of 15 to 1 (CBD:THC, 15:1) is achieved, it is a very short leap to reach a 30 to 1 ratio.

At the time of this writing, April 2014, Florida has just passed a law that allows the Charlotte's Web type medical MARIJUANA strains to be used for the treatment of epilepsy and cancer, as long as the THC content is below 0.8%. The Florida Senate passed the bill with a 30-9 vote on a Friday, and a day after the House supported it 111-7. Florida Governor Rick Scott has said he'll sign it.

If one does some research, they will see that cannabis was used as a propaganda tool back in the late 1930's and early 1940's by people with agendas. This book will not address these issues, but propaganda tools like the movie "Reefer Madness" released back in 1936 speak for themselves. If you haven't seen "Reefer Madness", it was a wildly over the top propaganda film designed to frighten naive, innocent minded people of the horrors of what smoking MARIJUANA can do to you. It was on par with a Frankenstein movie and by today's standards, absolutely ridiculous.[6]

It is really no surprise that the U.S. Pharmacopeia is loaded with medications that can be highly addictive. Addiction potential has not stopped many drugs from entering the market. If it had, there would not be nearly the amount of pain and anxiety medications we have available today, as many of them are addictive, as we all know.

As it Stands Now

Caffeine, alcohol and nicotine (coffee, booze and cigarettes) are all legal and all can be lethal in high enough doses. MARIJUANA is not, yet it is a Schedule 1 drug – the most dangerous classification.

MARIJUANA has even less addiction potential than caffeine and nicotine. Alcohol has been demonstrated to be worse in all categories across the addiction board than MARIJUANA, and alcohol can even be lethal in withdrawal.

By these standards, alcohol and cigarettes would surely qualify to be on the government's most dangerous drug list, would they not?

As a licensed registered nurse and as a member of the American Cannabis Nurses Association, my position on MARIJUANA is this: change the status of MARIJUANA from illegal to a legal medicinal status as it once was decades ago. Even though there is an addiction potential with MARIJUANA it is less addictive than cigarettes, alcohol and caffeine (coffee is served up all day long and sometimes free!).

We all have an endocannabinoid system. This system is just as vulnerable to disease and deficiency as any other system in the human body. The only plant in the world that has a direct therapeutic effect on this system is the cannabis family of plants. As it stands now, the cannabis plant is a Schedule 1 drug. In my opinion, there is enough pressure, both political and social, that a cannabis reclassification will happen. I could be wrong about this, but I hope not.

At least, right now, we have legal CBD, the second most recognized component of the cannabis plant. Research shows that CBD itself seems to be a medicinal in its own right. CBD has helped so many end their suffering and it is important to remember, in this light, that CBD and THC share the same molecular structure. These mother-nature-made molecules are here to help us, not harm us, as some would have you believe.

Time has a way of sifting out the truth. Looking back through history, along with recent discoveries, it is evident where the truth lies with the cannabis saga. The truth is that cannabis can alleviate people's suffering and is a major medicinal of our time. Our eyes have been opened. In light of the endocannabinoid system discovery and the cannabis plant cannabinoids, it is clearly time to move forward. Legalize, don't vilify, cannabis and medical MARIJUANA.

Chapter 6 References:

[1] Alcohol. Other Drugs and Health: Current Evidence
www.bu.edu/aodhealth/issues/issue_sept13/rastegar_dsm5.
html

[2] The National Cancer Institute at the National Institutes of
Health:
www.cancer.gov/cancertopics/pdq/cam/cannabis/patient/page2

[3] Office of Diversion Control:
www.deadiversion.usdoj.gov/schedules/

[4] Definition of Controlled Substance Schedules:
www.deadiversion.usdoj.gov/21cfr/cfr/2108cfrt.htm

[5] Charlotte's Web – CBD for Epilepsy:
www.youtube.com/watch?v=S9qkYLtAhSQ

[6] Reefer Madness:
www.youtube.com/watch?v=54xWo7ITFbg

References

American Cannabis Nurses Association website:
www.americancannabisnursesassociation.org

CBD Discounted and Alternative Health Products Coupon Code "CBD10" for 10% off CBD Products:
www.URparamount.com

Dr. Allan Frankel, MD, Greenbridge Medical, Santa Monica, CA

Website: www.greenbridgemed.com
YouTube: www.youtube.com/watch?v=2J7PaelhZwc

DISCLAIMER

These statements have not been evaluated by the Food and Drug Administration (FDA).

This information is not intended to diagnose, treat, cure, or prevent any disease.

Please note that the information in this book is for educational purposes only and is not meant as an alternative to medical diagnosis or treatment. The authors make no representations or warranties in relation to the health information in this book. If you think you may be suffering from any medical condition, you should seek medical attention. You should never delay seeking medical advice, disregard medical advice, or discontinue medical treatment because of information in this book. If you are considering making any changes to your lifestyle, diet or nutrition, you should consult with your doctor.

About the Authors

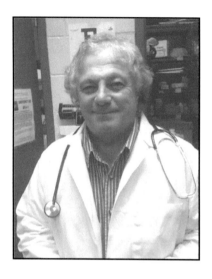

Dr. Steven Leonard-Johnson
RN-BC, PhD, LMT, BCB

Steve is a member of the American Cannabis Nurses Association (ACNA). He is certified as a Psychiatric and Mental Health Nurse by the American Nurses Credentialing Center. Steve has many years of experience working in the acute care psychiatric setting including the emergency room, geriatric, forensic, acute detox, adult, dual diagnosis and intensive care psychiatric units.

Steve has worked in New York metropolitan area hospitals and spent five years in home health care as a psychiatric nurse in an under-served, rural area of Maine.

Steve is also a Senior Fellow with the Biofeedback Certification International Alliance. Certified by the National Certification Board for Therapeutic Massage and Bodywork, Steve is an active member of the American Massage Therapy Association. His area of clinical interest is in the study of mind/body interaction preferring holistic treatment of pain, anxiety and trauma; he has developed a sophisticated style in deep tissue massage using CBD oil, infrared heat and high speed vibration as the base and he is writing about it in his next book, using his many years as a medical massage therapist as his guide.

Steve is an active member of
American Mensa and Intertel societies.

About the Co-Author
Editor & Graphic Artist

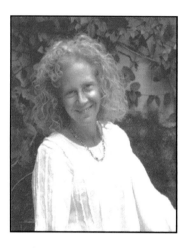

Tina Rappaport, BFA
Owner, www.URparamount.com

Tina has been researching alternative health for over 40 years, starting as a teenager, with the ultimate goal of overcoming lifelong joint problems. Head to toe, hands down, her health is much more vibrant than when she was half her age. She no longer walks with a cane or uses braces on her neck, hands or knees. Even severe lower back pain and neuralgia have faded away. Headaches are a thing of the past.

Over her lifetime, Tina has become quite knowledgeable in pH balancing, ionized water, raw foods, veganism, sprouting, dehydrating, energy medicine (frequency healing) and other alternative modalities.

After varying career paths including custom stained glass windows, grant writing for NYU's School of Education and video production and editing in her own business, Tina ventured into an online business selling products that support her health including water ionizers, the Rife 101 Energy System, Chlorella & Spirulina and other pH balancing and detox products. CBD is the most recent addition.

Readers of this book are eligible to receive a 10% discount on already discounted CBD product prices at www.URparamount.com – use coupon code "CBD10" at checkout.

"My mission is to help you...

...because, YOU ARE paramount!"